I0837534

A NEW NORMAL

Practical Living Tips for Staying Healthy in an Unhealthy World

By
Goldie Kirkbride

Copyright © 2020 Goldie Kirkbride
All rights reserved.

Introduction

As I write this, one cannot get through a single day without hearing about the rising death toll from COVID 19. It has been deemed a global pandemic, and whole countries have come to a screeching halt in efforts to avoid spreading infection. Here in the U.S.A. employees in "essential" jobs such as healthcare, food production, sanitation, and transportation of necessary goods are working to keep fellow citizens fed and taken care of; those who can work from home are dependent on communications technology to continue earning a paycheck, and those who fall into other categories have been told to stay home. Economies have taken a huge hit world-wide, and the virus does not care what demographic one is in; it has killed paupers and celebrities alike.

This book is intended to give you practical tips on how to minimize your chances of falling ill from this or any of the myriad other germs you encounter on a daily basis.

Inside these pages, I will give you practical advice on how to avoid "catching something" in public or at work as well as how to combat an invasion in your own home.

As an IIN Certified Health Coach, a volunteer First Aid Responder, and with over a decade of experience in a food processing plant where good sanitation practices are not only imperative for food safety's sake, but required by law, I have learned how to keep myself and others as safe as possible. I am also a mother and a grandmother, so I know that it is not always easy or possible to avoid sick people or get them to cooperate with what is best for them.

This book will help you find some measures that you can implement with immediate results for everyday life, and you will also find some advice that is an investment in your future health.

I changed my Standard American Diet to a more nutrient dense version about two years ago. The result is fewer sick days, less severe illness when "something is going around", and fewer aches and pains. I am not on any prescriptions either, which is a win in my opinion. The food processing companies I have worked for have proven that proper sanitation methods can prevent pathogens from getting into consumer products, and I have learned to modify their processes to fit into my home life.

Please do not set this book aside until later. Feel free to skip around. Find a tip that you can do now, and take the first step to protecting yourself and your loved ones.

The information in these pages is not meant to diagnose or treat any illness. My advice is not a substitute for that of a medical professional. If you are sick, seek medical help. No one can be 100% safe from illness, but you can make a huge impact on the level of germs and contamination that your body must contend with, starting today.

CHAPTER 1: GERMS. WHAT ARE THEY, ANYWAY?

Germs are everywhere, and many of them can make us sick. However, not all germs are alike, and knowing thy enemy is half the battle, as the saying goes.

Germs can be bacteria, spirochetes, viruses, parasites, or fungi. At any given time, we are probably hosting germs from each classification.

Put simply, bacteria are living things in the plant family. Spirochetes are a corkscrew-shaped microbe. Viruses are not considered living creatures because they cannot reproduce on their own. Parasites feed off of the host. Fungi are in the vegetable kingdom but have no chlorophyll with which to make their own food.

Bacteria

Not all bacteria are bad. The human digestive system relies on good bacteria to break down our food and to contribute to our immune systems. The bad ones commonly cause diarrhea, ear infections, and respiratory infections, or even death in some cases.

- o Handwashing with regular soap and water and good personal hygiene can physically remove the bacteria from your skin. Anti-bacterial soaps and cleaners can kill them on hands and surfaces.
- o See Appendix A for handwashing tips.

Antibiotics are used to kill bacteria. The problem with these products is that they are not selective in which bacteria they kill, so the good ones are killed along with the bad ones.

- o If you are prescribed a course of antibiotics, take all of them as directed so all of the bad ones are eradicated, not just the weak ones, and take a probiotic to replenish your good bacteria. Stopping antibiotics too soon can contribute to the development of "superbugs" which are antibiotic resistant.

Spirochetes

Spirochetes can be harmless, but a well-known pathogenic one causes syphilis, one of several venereal diseases. Others cause skin lesions. The best prevention is to avoid sexual contact with strangers; many people can be asymptomatic (not showing signs of illness), and transmit the pathogen to others, including an infant during childbirth.

- o Good personal hygiene is imperative to avoiding this kind of infection.
- o Abstain from sex or choose a monogamous partner who tests negative for STDs.
- o Wear condoms with non-oxynol 9 to reduce the chance of transmission.

Viruses

Viruses cause problems because they invade like something out of a science fiction movie and hi-jack the host's cells to replicate themselves. These pathogens are like a missing link in the development of life because they contain RNA, a genetic material inferior to DNA, which cannot reproduce itself without commandeering a living cell and using its capabilities to produce virus proteins. The host cells are destroyed in the process. Different viruses tend to favor particular types of cells because their protein shell must "fit" the host cell's receptors. The shapes of viruses range from spiky to geometric, which is why our immune systems may struggle to recognize the enemy and produce antibodies for a specific invader. Viruses are smaller than other microbes, so they can pass through certain filters and barriers that would stop a bacterium or parasite. Therefore, distancing oneself from known sick people is the best defense there is.

Antibiotics do not work against a virus. Keeping antibiotics from your last prescription to take for your next illness may not work and can contribute to "superbugs."

If you have been bitten by an animal, seek immediate medical treatment because rabies is deadly. I found out that the old advice to capture the animal for testing to avoid having to get the series of shots to prevent rabies in the victim is useless; my daughter was bitten by a raccoon in our chicken coup. I shot the raccoon, but none of the health authorities were interested in testing the carcass, nor could they refer me to anyone who could.

Viral infection treatments are mostly geared toward providing comfort from symptoms and supporting the body while it works to ward off the infection.

- o Vaccinations are available.

It is my opinion that too many vaccines are given at once, and the contaminants in them can be dangerous. Research the ingredients in vaccines before you agree to them. Polysorbate 80 moves contaminants through the blood/brain barrier that would not otherwise get in; it is a preservative used in vaccines with more than one microbe, such as three-in-one shots. Thimerosal is a compound containing mercury. Aluminum is included to heighten the body's immune response. Furthermore, vaccine microbes are "cultured," or grown, in tissue from animals or aborted fetuses. Consider your religious beliefs and personal values before accepting vaccination.

- Wash hands frequently with soap and water.
- Use hand sanitizers if hand washing is not available.
- Stay at least six feet away from people; that is about how far a cough or sneeze can carry germs.
- Seek medical attention if you have a fever over 100° F, severe cough or sore throat, or severe intestinal issues.

Parasites

Parasites include worms and protozoa.

Worms reproduce with eggs and imbed themselves in the host, usually in the intestinal tract, and feed off the host. Worms can enter through the skin or by ingestion or inhalation, usually from contaminated soil or water.

- Wear shoes and gloves if digging dirt that may be contaminated with fecal matter.
- Worm eggs can be inhaled or swallowed. Thoroughly cook foods to kill both eggs and worms.

Malaria parasites reproduce inside of the host's cells, destroying the cell when they break out. This parasite is transmitted through mosquito bites.

- Use of mosquito netting and repellants can help prevent infection.
- Restrict travel to areas of the world where malaria is common.

Toxoplasmosis is a parasitic infection that causes mild symptoms in adults but can cause birth defects of the nervous system in an infected fetus.

- Pregnant women should avoid contact with cat feces because the protozoan can be harbored in the feline intestinal tract.
- Thoroughly cook foods, especially meats.

Fungi

Fungi include molds, yeast, mushrooms, toadstools, and the like. Obviously, some mushrooms are edible while some are deadly if ingested, so not all fungi are bad either. Candida albicans is the most common example of a fungal infection in humans. It infects the skin or mucous membranes and is the cause of the infamous vaginal yeast infection, but men can get it too, and are often guilty of transferring it between partners.

Most fungi prefer warm, damp, dark areas.

- o Practice good hygiene including handwashing, showering, and wearing clean clothes.
- o Allow natural light and air into rooms when possible.
- o Use the exhaust fan in the bathroom during baths or showers to remove excess humidity wherein mildew thrives.
- o Use a dehumidifier to dry out damp areas where mildew and mold like to grow.

Chapter Summary/Key Takeaways

Knowing what to expect in your environment can help you avoid these germs, and if you do "catch something," you can better focus your countermeasures to eradicate the enemy. The treatment for one type of germ probably won't work for another, so if you are ill, it is best to seek medical diagnosis to identify which pathogen is attacking you and what to do to fight the invasion. Avoiding an infection in the first place is always preferable. In the next chapter, you will learn more about how to avoid infections by keeping the microbes away or killing them.

CHAPTER 2: STOP THE INVASION

If you wanted to prevent criminals from invading your home, how would you begin? You might start by installing locks on doors and windows, eliminating hiding places so they cannot sneak up on you, and having an alarm system installed. If the bad guys still try to break in, you might call for help while defending yourself with whatever weapons you have on hand until the trained police arrive.

Your body does pretty much the same thing with a germ invasion. In a best-case scenario, the microbes are blocked before they ever get inside your body. If they do make it in, your body defends itself until the trained "army" of antibodies, white blood cells, and/or t-cells is mustered.

Methods of Transmission

From whence do they come?

The enemy travels by different routes. Successful defense requires knowledge of how they move and how to block them.

Airborne pathogens travel via the airways. When an infected person sneezes or coughs, tiny droplets of saliva, mucus, and the germs they contain are atomized into the air up to about six feet away. A passerby may inhale those droplets through his nose or mouth. Those droplets can also land on other people or objects and survive for a few minutes or several days.

- o Sneeze or cough into a tissue, handkerchief, or your sleeve. This reduces how far the droplets travel, and it also avoids getting the germ-laden snot on your hands to be transferred to everything you touch.

Some germs are transmitted through casual contact. Whether they originated from a sneeze or a handshake, people can pass along the bad guys without being aware of it. For example, imagine an infected person with a runny nose sneezes into a tissue, then throws the tissue into the trash. What is wrong with that, you ask? That person then opens the door to the restroom to go wash his hands. Those germs are potentially on the handle to the restroom door, so the next person who grabs that handle to enter the restroom could be picking up hitchhiking germs. If he rubs his eyes or nose, those germs are now in! A break in the skin, contaminated hands touching eyes, nose, or mouth, or sex can all be an unlocked door for the invaders.

o   Using a tissue and washing hands are great, but not 100% effective. Keep practicing good hygiene because it reduces the pathogen load that your body must fight.

Sexually transmitted diseases (STDs) are the subject of many jokes, but they are no laughing matter. Herpes, HIV, HPV, chlamydia, or yeast infections are a few of the diseases that are transmitted through sexual contact.

o   Condoms can reduce the incidence of transfer of pathogens from one person to another, but they are not 100% effective. Some microbes can pass through the material.

Body fluids of a person or animal should be treated as biohazardous material. Mucus, saliva, urine, feces, or blood can all carry diseases. Insects or animals, including the human animal, can transmit pathogens through bites (rabies, West Nile disease, Lyme disease, malaria).

o   See Appendix B for how to handle biohazards.
o   For bites, wash the affected area thoroughly with soap and water. In the case of wildlife bites or strange domestic animals, seek medical attention immediately; rabies is one disease that does not present symptoms until it is too late for medical treatments to stop the illness.
o   Smaller wounds can be treated with triple antibiotic ointment, an antiseptic spray, or tea tree oil. If you believe bodily fluids of an infected person or a stranger have been ingested, aspirated, or have contacted your broken skin or gotten in your eyes, seek medical attention. Physicians can do testing to determine if you have been exposed to any pathogens.
o   For puncture wounds, such as splinters or nails that poke deeply, see a doctor about preventing tetanus.

Just getting body fluids or a germ on you does not always mean you will contract the disease. As long as you keep it out of your body, or at least limit your exposure to levels your body can ward off, you can come into contact with the germs but not get sick. This is particularly important to remember, because you can carry those germs around, transfer them to someone more vulnerable than you, and infect them without knowing you ever had it. These safety tips are not just for you; they also protect others around you.

Defensive Tactics

So, how do you stop the invaders from making it inside?

Your skin is your first line of defense. It is a physical barrier between your body and the outside world full of potentially harmful factors, be they germs, allergens, or pollution. Handwashing is the number one way to avoid the contaminants from getting inside your body.

While you are doing your part to "lock the doors," the "police" are on patrol, often taking care of invaders without your knowing the germs were ever there.

- o Regular soap and water serve to physically remove dirt (a hiding place) and pathogens.
- o Antibacterial soaps combat bacteria and E2 soaps kill both bacteria and viruses.
- o Wash hands after using the restroom, before and after caring for a sick person, after removing exam or cleaning gloves, after touching contact surfaces, after smoking, after assisting children with the potty, before and after eating, before and after preparing or processing food or beverages, before and after work tasks, after gardening, after petting or handling animals, or any time you may pick up or transfer contaminants.
- o See Appendix A for proper handwashing techniques.

Using antibacterial and antiviral soaps and gels continuously can create "superbugs" by killing off the weak germs and leaving the stronger ones to survive and reproduce. Resort to using these weapons if the following apply:

- o You have health problems that compromise your immune system.
- o When illness is running rampant or someone you live or work closely with is sick. these products are a good idea.
- o If you handle food or beverages for others' consumption, by all means, use sanitizers.
- o Use hand sanitizers if handwashing is not available or if you are sick so that you avoid giving the germs to others.

Frequent handwashing can irritate the skin and even cause dryness and cracking. Having dry cracked skin is similar to having a cut; cuts, cracks, and punctures are all entry points for invaders.

- o Use moisturizers to help prevent dry, cracked skin.
- o Staying hydrated helps your skin remain supple naturally.

Surgical masks (N95), face shields, and exam gloves are the benchmark for keeping healthcare workers safe when in contact with potentially infected patients as well as keeping their germs from reaching a vulnerable patient. These masks are not necessary for the average person because we are not in a position of encountering elevated numbers of disease-stricken individuals. In times of low demand, it wouldn't be a bad idea to buy a box or two to keep on hand in your preparedness supplies, but hoarding the masks and gloves during an epidemic means that there will be short supply for medical professionals to protect themselves while trying to help the ill. Another thing to consider is that these supplies do not last indefinitely. If you decide to keep some around for a future epidemic, then be sure to rotate your stock from time to time because materials eventually deteriorate.

- o Wearing masks is a voluntary precaution when ill, susceptible to illness, or during epidemics.
- o Cloth masks are an alternative to the disposable ones. They may prevent an infected person from sneezing or coughing large amounts of a contagion out into the environment, but they are not likely to prevent microbes from the environment from reaching one entirely; they simply are not able to filter to that level. If you would like to wear one, go to www.cdc.gov in the U.S.A. for directions on how to make, wear, and care for a cloth mask, or they can be found online for purchase.

Your nose and bronchial tubes are lined with cilia, hair-like structures that trap or sweep microbes out. Your respiratory tract also produces mucus to trap and wash out irritants. A cough or sneeze propels the invaders out of the body. This is why fully suppressing a cough is not a good thing in most cases.

- o Using an expectorant to thin mucus and make it easier to expel may prove helpful. Use according to the label instructions or contact your physician before using.
- o Maintaining a physical distance from others of at least six feet (two average adults' arm-lengths), otherwise known as "social distancing," can significantly reduce the rate of transmission between people. You cannot catch a bug if it never reaches you.
- o Avoid handshaking, sharing utensils or tools, and contacting common surfaces such as handles, buttons, or ink pens.

Killing germs on hard surfaces can slow or stop the spread of pathogens. Remember, you cannot clean anything if your tools are dirty. Use of rubber gloves is recommended for chemical use.

- For a list of EPA registered cleaners with anti-viral properties, go to https://www.epa.gov/pesticide-registration/list-n-disinfectants-use-against-sars-cov-2 .
- Thorough cleaning with regular cleansers and water can physically remove germs.
- Use of anti-bacterial and anti-viral products constantly can contribute to "superbugs." Save this arsenal for when someone is sick.
- Rubbing alcohol ($\geq 70\%$), chlorine bleach, bleach cleaners, anti-bacterial cleaners, and spray disinfectants are examples of products that can reduce the number of germs in your home or workplace.
- Wash dishes and utensils soon after use.
- Dishwasher-safe items should be washed in the dishwasher because it can use higher temperatures than your hands can safely withstand.
- Allow hand-washed items to air dry to avoid spreading leftover germs with the towel. You can also choose to air-dry dishes in the dishwasher by opening the door and pulling the racks out. Remember to remove any sharp or breakable objects if you have small children in the home.
- Launder cleaning cloths or towels after each use during illnesses or epidemics.
- It is the opinion of this author that sponges harbor too many bacteria to be reused at all. Put them through a dishwasher cycle or soak them in a bleach solution if you must reuse sponges.
- Dedicate floor care items for the floor only.
- Dedicate bathroom cleaning tools and gloves for the bathroom only.
- Apply disinfectants and cleaners from bottom to top on upright surfaces so the fresh chemicals contact the surface being cleaned. Also, applying chemicals from top to bottom may cause streaking.
- Rinse vertical surfaces top to bottom to flush soils down and away.
- Do not use spray hoses on drains; the splashing can contaminate the surrounding surfaces you already cleaned. Use a brush that is dedicated only to drains.

- o Whatever cleaners you choose to use, do not mix chlorine bleach or chlorinated bleach cleaners with ammonia or other chemicals. You can create lethal poisonous gases. Read labels for proper dilution and use.
- o Color-coding reusable cleaning supplies can help avoid cross-contamination. Perhaps you have a blue bucket for washing down walls, but you have a black bucket for floors. Whatever colors you choose, be consistent so others do not get confused.
- o Rinse reusable cleaning supplies and air dry after use.
- o See Appendix C for cleaning checklists.

Laundry is another task that can benefit the war on illness.

- o Wash bed linens at least once per week, more frequently for a sick person.
- o Wash laundry on the hottest setting that the fabrics can endure.
- o Use bleach on whites.
- o Tumble dry durable fabrics on high heat.
- o Delicate fabrics can be tumble dried on low heat, but they need to be heated for a longer period to be sanitized.

Ultraviolet light kills many germs. That is why it is used everywhere from food processing plants to aerated septic systems.

- o If you live in an area where you can hang your laundry out on a clothesline, take advantage of the sun's ultraviolet germ-fighting superpowers.
- o Open curtains and blinds to allow sunlight into your home or workplace to work its magic.
- o Try to get at least ten minutes of exposure to direct sunlight every day to boost your immune system with vitamin-D production.

Unless you have skin cancer or photosensitivity, you do not need to be afraid of a little bit of sunshine. Excessive sensitivity may be caused by retinol skin creams, birth control pills, or other prescriptions, so if you use these products, limit your unprotected sun exposure. Gardeners or landscapers should be aware that contact with some plants can create photosensitivity. Sunblock does negate the benefits of sun exposure, so supplemental vitamin-D may be helpful, but let your physician know what you are taking to avoid drug interactions or overdosing. That being said, baking until you burn is a terrible idea; a sunburn is radiation damage. Use some common sense when it comes to how long to be outdoors without shade or around the water when you aren't used to it, and keep in mind that the sun's rays reflected off of the water can burn you even if you are in the shade of a canopy or umbrella.

The hydrochloric acid in your stomach destroys many germs that enter the digestive tract, but it is not foolproof, so do not ignore what is getting in through your digestive system.

- o The three-second rule is not a thing. Germs (and whatever else has been tracked into the area on shoes or pets) will get on dropped food immediately.
- o Thoroughly cook meats to kill pathogens. Most microbes are killed once the center of the piece of meat has reached 140° F. If you do not have a meat thermometer, cook until the thickest part of the food is no longer pink, and the juices run clear.
- o Cooked foods must be held above 140° to prevent bacterial growth. Refrigerate leftovers immediately. Any cooked food left at room temperature should be thrown out after four hours.
- o Cold foods should be kept below 40° F on ice or in the refrigerator. Any refrigerated foods not kept cold should be thrown out after four hours
- o Wash vegetables and fruits, even if you are going to peel them. The knife can carry any germs or pollutants from the surface into the flesh.
- o Store foods properly. The refrigerator should be kept at 40° F. A deep freeze should be kept at 0° F.
- o Large quantities of food should be portioned before freezing or refrigerating so they will reach target temperatures faster.
- o Store refrigerated raw meats in the bottom-most compartment, never above ready-to-eat foods.
- o Clean surfaces and utensils after contacting raw meat.
- o Wash your hands after handling raw meats.
- o Do NOT use the same knife and cutting board for raw meats and for vegetables that will not be cooked. For example, cut up rinsed vegetables first, then cut up raw meat. You could also use separate cutting boards.

Good personal hygiene is mandatory. None of your efforts at cleaning the home or avoiding germs will work if you are a walking Petri dish.

Body odor is caused by bacteria flourishing in sweat or in moist genital areas. Bad breath is usually bacteria colonizing the mouth and gums, although it can be an underlying health issue.

- o Shower or bathe at least once per day, preferably before bedtime.
- o Use deodorants and/or antiperspirants on underarms.
- o Brush teeth twice a day at a minimum.
- o See Appendix E for personal hygiene guidelines.

Showering and washing your hair physically remove microbes and allergens along with sweat, dirt or gross soils where germs thrive. If you like to shower in the morning to wake up and freshen up, that's fine, but showering when you get home from work, a workout, or outdoor play can prevent insects, parasites, microbes and allergens from being distributed throughout your home.

Floss, brush, and rinse teeth and gums to break up bacterial colonies in the mouth. At least brush your teeth after meals. Change your toothbrush every three months whether the bristles look worn or not; that is the time it takes for the bacteria to build troublesome colonies.

- o Remove shoes at the door to avoid carrying dirt, allergens, and microbes through the home.
- o Bathe pets regularly or use a grooming service to reduce allergens and parasites.
- o To avoid transferring worms, do not let animals lick your child's or your hands or face.
- o Teach children not to share clothing, hats, or combs and brushes at school or daycare where they could be infested by lice or bed bugs from other kids.

Chapter Summary/Key Takeaways

Now you know that pathogens are transmitted via air, direct contact with infected people or animals, contact with contaminated surfaces, sexual contact, body fluids, or inhalation and ingestion.

Handwashing, housekeeping, laundry, sanitizing surfaces, and physical distancing are possible ways of avoiding catching germs.

In the next chapter, you will learn what to do if you get sick despite your best prevention efforts.

CHAPTER 3: WHAT TO DO WHEN YOU ARE SICK

So, you tried your best to keep the invaders outside, but somehow, they managed to find their way in. It is time to call the police, but you need to defend yourself until they apprehend the perpetrators. How can you minimize the damage until the bad guys can be eradicated?

What You Can Do Now

Okay. You know you are coming down with something. What comes next?

- o Take your temperature. Anything above 100° F. rates a visit with a physician.
- o Many physicians offer virtual visits to avoid a waiting room and an office full of germs to share. Call ahead to learn whether your doctor can do a phone or video consultation with you and how much it will cost.
- o If you are coughing or sneezing, wear a mask if you have one. Check in with the receptionist. You may be asked to wait in a separate area from the less contagious patients, and many doctors will get you in faster to minimize germ sharing.
- o Let your physician know all of the medications and supplements you take to avoid possible interactions with prescriptions he may decide are indicated for your current illness.
- o Always remind your doctor if you have any allergies, even if you have had the same doctor for years.
- o If you are prescribed medications, get them as soon as possible, and take them exactly as directed.
- o Do not forget to call off of work to avoid spreading germs to coworkers or customers.
- o Ask your doctor for an excuse slip if your employer requires it.
- o Seek a second opinion if you have any doubts about your doctor's diagnosis or prognosis.
- o Understand placebo and nocebo effects. Placebo is your mental and physical improvement without any real medical intervention. Nocebo is your mental and physical deterioration simply because you were told to expect it. Both are well documented, so feel free to look these effects up for yourself.

At home, there are some other things you can do to be more comfortable, speed your recovery, and avoid giving the illness to your loved ones or roommates.

- If possible, isolate yourself or the sick person to one bedroom and one bathroom.
- The sick person should avoid handling food or dishes for others.
- If there is a young child in the household, someone who is not sick should take care of the child and keep him occupied away from the convalescent.
- Washing hands is as relevant as ever.
- Contact surfaces must be kept clean and sanitized. Keep a can of disinfectant handy, but make sure it is out of reach of small children.
- Drink plenty of fluids. Hydration is imperative to allow the body to operate properly and to flush away wastes.
- Eat lightly. Emphasize fruits and vegetables. Heavy protein and fat meals just add to the work the body is doing while one is ill. Lay off the sugary confections.
- If you like tea, now is the time to indulge frequently. Several herbal teas can be helpful; look for blends that are targeted for your particular symptoms. Also, many plants used for teas have antiviral and anti-inflammatory or immune-boosting properties. One example is peppermint tea, which soothes nausea.
- Let the sunshine in unless you are sensitive to light. It helps one's morale as well as being a germ fighter.
- If weather allows, get some fresh air by opening a window or stepping out on a porch.
- If you have congestion or a cough, a vaporizer near the chair or bed may be helpful.
- An expectorant, or mucus thinner, may help if you are "plugged up" or if the mucus is hard to bring up from the lungs and feels as if it is choking you.
- Eating chicken noodle soup is a tried-and-true standby for good reason. You can also just drink broth if you are not feeling up to solid foods.
- If tissues are needed, I highly recommend the kind with lotion to protect your nose from abrasion.
- I hope you have plenty of toilet paper available in case of diarrhea.
- If the illness is highly contagious, use disposable plates and flatware if possible. Wash regular dishes and utensils in a dishwasher or in soapy water with a little bleach (use the

amount recommended on the container's dilution directions. For the latter, you may want to use some clean household rubber gloves to avoid drying out the skin. Make sure the gloves you use for dishwashing have not been used to clean anything else.

Chapter Summary/Key Takeaways

Remember, if you or someone in your household is sick with something contagious, isolate that person as much as possible and keep everything disinfected.

If you are caring for a sick person with a contagious illness, protect yourself with a facemask, disposable latex or nitrile gloves, and cleanliness. Make sure the patient takes any medications on time, has plenty of fluids to drink, and is as comfortable as can be. It is easier for them and for you if you place a supply of tissues, drinks, crackers, and a remote or reading material within reach.

If you are the sick person, be considerate of others. Cover your mouth and nose when coughing or sneezing, wash hands frequently, practice the best hygiene you can muster the energy for, and avoid touching common contact items whenever possible.

Coming up in the next chapter, I will give you some tips you can put into practice for a long-term approach to overall wellness. After all, it is preferable not to get sick in the first place.

CHAPTER 4: SUPPORT YOUR IMMUNE SYSTEM

Take a long-term approach to wellness.

How does your body get rid of pathogens, and how can you support it in the process?

Anytime your body encounters a foreign body, which can be anything that is not recognized as part of your own body, the immune system must decide if the entity is friend or foe.

Allergies are your body's overreaction to something that it perceives as a threat. If your allergies are anything but a minor annoyance, then seek medical advice. For minor allergies, avoidance of allergens or use of OTC medications will probably suffice.

I am going to focus on what you can do to make your immune system strong and minimize the load on your body's defenses. A strong immune system can quickly identify pathogens and has the resources to efficiently kill the enemy.

Diet

When one hears the word "diet," weight loss usually comes to mind for most people. While maintaining a reasonable weight is helpful for overall health, what I am referring to here is your everyday style of eating.

Whatever your dietary preference, be it omnivorous, vegan, or something in between, your body needs certain vitamins, minerals, and amino acids to build and maintain cells. The closer your foods are to their natural state, the better, except for raw meats. Many of the good qualities of a food are destroyed by heat or offset by added sugars and unhealthful fats.

- o Eat a wide variety of foods in a rainbow of colors (not artificial ones) to maximize the range of nutrients you are getting.
- o Choose the less processed version of a plant-based food, most of the time. An orange is better than orange juice. A cherry is better than cherry pie.
- o Eat healthful foods rather than taking supplements, when possible. A salad of leafy greens and your favorite crudités is preferable to some bottled powder of plants that have no life left in them.
- o Consult a dietitian or nutritionist for specific plans for you based on dietary preferences, health conditions, or medications.

Other general diet tips for keeping your body humming along regularly follow:

- o Stay hydrated. I say that a lot because it is important. It is possible to overdo it, but that is rare.
- o Cook meats to kill common pathogens.
- o Avoid foods that trigger your allergies or sensitivities. For example, if you are lactose-intolerant, you are better off avoiding dairy foods than to continue eating them while popping dairy aid pills.
- o Limit sugar. Sugars feed bacteria, and you can count on them being the bad ones. Sugars also cause insulin spikes, which can set you up to get a fatty liver or Type II diabetes. I believe it is no coincidence that people with these health conditions are more prone to developing cancers or succumbing to pathogens.
- o Maintain a weight in your doctor's recommended range. Excess fat causes strain on every part of you from the circulatory system to the joints. Fat also produces estrogen, which can feed certain cancers.
- o Drink water, not calories. Sugary drinks, juices, and alcoholic beverages add empty calories, or calories without significant nutrition.
- o Go for nutrient dense foods. That means making a more nutritious choice for the calories you consume. For example, you can munch on raw vegetables to your heart's content; they are full of vitamins, minerals, antioxidants, and fiber among other things. Eating a bag of miniature candy bars will leave you craving more and has very little nutritive value.
- o Wash fruits and vegetables whether they are conventionally grown or organic. Unless you grew them yourself, you do not really know who or what has touched your food.
- o Avoid processed meats and packaged goods full of preservatives.
- o Avoid artificial colors, flavors, and dyes. There are enough chemicals contaminating our environments without eating more of them.
- o Sugar-free products may be a favorite of diabetics and chronic dieters, but they are a scientific marvel of chemical engineering.
- o Eat foods with anti-viral properties, such as garlic and onion.
- o Eat foods with anti-bacterial properties, such as honey.

Supplements

The Standard American Diet (SAD) is full of processed, convenient foods. What American kid has not eaten macaroni and cheese from a box dinner kit along with a hot dog? There is not a lot of nutrition in those. Even if you try to feed your family plenty of fruits and vegetables, canned, frozen, or fresh, our soils are depleted from decades of relentless, intensive farming. Typical fertilizers list three constituents: Nitrogen, Phosphorus, and Potassium. There are far more trace minerals that are important to our health, but they just are not being put back into the soil.

Our bodies depend on having the correct raw materials in sufficient quantities to grow, repair, and defend our physical integrity.

Taking a multi-vitamin can be a boon to most people in the general population. It is somewhat complicated to choose specific supplements, and overdosing on a vitamin can be toxic.

As a rule of thumb, water soluble vitamins will not build up in the body while fat-soluble vitamins can accumulate, especially in body fat, which is where the body tends to store excess anything.

If you want to take supplements, working with a nutritionist or dietician is a good place to start.

In my opinion, taking supplements that your body is supposed to be making on its own is a license for your body to quit manufacturing that vitamin or hormone. A widely consumed supplement is melatonin. Melatonin is naturally made in the pineal gland in the brain. Using a synthetic version may cause your pineal gland to stop producing this hormone because it thinks you have a sufficient level (which is artificially raised.) If you have had severe head trauma and cannot produce it, then take a supplement. Otherwise, do some research and find out what your body needs to produce an adequate supply on its own. In this case, melatonin production is triggered by your Circadian rhythm, darkness, and quiet. Avoid stress, artificial light, and stimulants before bedtime.

- o Consume or take a probiotic. These are the good guys. The more of them that become established in your digestive tract, the less room there is for the bad guys. Yogurt, kefir, and fermented foods are natural sources.
- o Consume or take prebiotics. These are the food for your probiotics. The same vegetables that you should already be eating are good for feeding your gut flora.

Pollutants, Contaminants, and Chemicals

The U.S.A. tends to lag far behind European countries when it comes to outlawing food additives and pesticides or controlling food ingredients. Brominated vegetable oil is used in popular sodas here in the U.S., but it is banned in Europe due to neurological effects.

Glyphosate is a well-known herbicide that pervades our food supply. Just because you do not hear about Monsanto anymore, do not assume the problem has gone away; Bayer bought them out.

What do pesticides and pollution have to do with your immune system? All contaminants add a workload to your body. Think of it this way: if you were spending a day cleaning your car interior and exterior, waxing and polishing away, you would probably have no problem handling it. Now a bird flies over and leaves you a present. Now you must drag the hose back out, but there is not any water coming out. While your back is turned, a cat walks across your freshly polished hood. Now you have to go back and wipe away the pawprints, but you do not have a clean chamois. You may begin to feel stressed, and what happened to the water supply anyway? Every extra, unnecessary task that gets piled on you makes you tired and depletes your resources.

Search the Internet for the effects of pesticides on human health, and you will get far more information than you may want to see. They can physically damage your body, causing anything from a sore throat to severe respiratory issues. Many are endocrine inhibitors which may contribute to autism and diabetes.

Air pollution can affect the respiratory tract, water pollution can poison your whole body, and heavy metal pollution in the ground can end up in your food.

The more chemicals in the food, the more processes in the body are taxed and confused by the extra chemicals.

If the body is busy trying to flush out contaminants, then it is using resources: fuel, water, and repair materials. Now, while your system is tired, along comes a virus. Your secret service bodyguards try to fight back with antibodies and white blood cells. If you have been using your resources to clear away pollution, now there are no building materials for the army of cells you need.

Everything is connected.

So, what can you do about it if it is in the food supply?
- o   Wash fruits and vegetables before peeling, cutting, or eating.
- o   Use a water filter for your drinking water.

- o Read labels and avoid ingredients with their chemical names. If it is not a food, vitamin, or mineral, then what is it doing in your food?
- o Grow some of your own foods. At least you will be able to control what chemicals you put on the plants or feed your animals.
- o Buy from a local farmers' market. When you can talk directly to someone who is producing your food, you can ask questions about how it was produced.

Chapter Summary/Key Takeaways

What you fuel your body with limits or supports your immune system. Avoid contaminants that overload your body's defense mechanisms.

CONCLUSION

I hope that I have given you some practical ideas to implement in your life to protect yourself and support natural healing and a strong immune system. Based on my personal experience and study of various topics, the information herein is true and factual to the best of my knowledge. I highly encourage you to read everything you can find about a particular topic and make your own decision about its applicability to your situation. Knowledge is power; sometimes it is just as important to know which questions to ask as it is to have the answers.

The information I have given in this publication is not meant to substitute for professional medical or psychological advice. If you have a medical or mental condition or suicidal or homicidal thoughts, seek professional care immediately. You can always seek a second opinion if you are not sure about one doctor's diagnosis or prognosis.

In the Appendixes, I have added some checklists and more thorough explanations for some key topics.

I hope my advice contributes positively to the quality of your life. Stay well.

APPENDIXES

Appendix A

Handwashing

Handwashing is one of the simplest, yet one of the most neglected methods for avoiding infectious diseases. Even those who wash their hands regularly rarely do a thorough job of it. Learn to do the following, and teach children to do the same to remove or reduce common contaminants from being carried into the body.

- Wet hands, preferably under running water.
- Use regular soap and water under normal circumstances. If illness is "going around" or if you have rendered first aid to someone, use antibacterial or E2 soap when it is available.
- Apply soap to hands. Rub and lather from wrists to fingertips, between fingers, and under nails. Continue lathering for at least twenty seconds. If you sing the "Happy Birthday" song twice, you will have reached twenty seconds.
- Rinse under running water, with hands pointed downward, so water rinses away the microbes and soap from wrists to fingertips.
- Dry with a towel or air dryer, from wrists to fingertips.

It is certainly possible that an emergency situation will catch one without any handwashing supplies available. Sawdust or dirt can be used to remove some of the fluids, but take care not to abrade your skin, which could create an entry point for pathogens

Appendix B

Biohazardous Waste

Biohazardous waste is anything from the body that could potentially be contaminated, and anything that has come into contact with such materials. It could include mucous, blood, saliva, vaginal secretions, semen, urine, feces, or any other tissue or fluid that could be contaminated with microbes.

A bandage is biohazardous material, although we rarely give it much thought. However, if you were to find a used bandage on the ground or floor, picking it up with your bare hands is inadvisable.

Treat all secretions and tissues as hazardous.

Small amounts of such waste can go in the regular garbage in the home setting. Put used bandages or wound dressings inside of a trash bag and tie it up when disposing.

Hypodermic needles, such as those used for diabetic care, should go in a sharps container to avoid puncturing the trash bag and anyone or animal who could come into contact with it. Contact your local county public health department to learn where to responsibly dispose of sharps containers. Some medical supply services offer a mail back service to dispose of the sharps you buy from them.

Before giving first aid or caring for someone where contact with body fluids is possible, protect yourself from biohazards. In an emergency, always call or have someone call 9-1-1 in the U.S.A.

- o Use exam gloves, not cleaning gloves, if available. Exam gloves are higher density. Other clean, waterproof gloves are better than nothing if you do not have exam gloves.
- o If performing rescue breathing, use a CPR mask if available. People in cardiac arrest will usually vomit, and without a mask, you risk getting vomit in your mouth.
- o A face shield or safety glasses would be well-advised if there is a chance that fluids could splatter or spray, but that obviously is not going to be commonly available in an emergency situation.
- o Wear an N95 facemask, if available, to avoid inhaling pathogens.

When cleaning up after contacting potentially hazardous bio-waste, consider the following tips:

- o   Dispose of any soiled bandages or materials in tied trash bag. If your workplace or facility requires it, use a red bio-hazard bag.
- o   Consider disposing of contaminated clothing, or launder on hottest settings.
- o   Use chlorine bleach on hard surfaces. Allow the bleach to sit on the surface for ten minutes. Rinse with water. If other cleaners are going to be used, make sure that you do not mix cleaners with bleach. Rinse the surface with water after the cleaner has sat long enough according to the package directions.
- o   Remove gloves correctly. See Appendix F for proper use of gloves
- o   WASH YOUR HANDS. If other skin was exposed, wash that too.
- o   If you think you may have inhaled, ingested, or been exposed to potential pathogens via eyes or compromised skin, contact your physician immediately.

Appendix C

Cleaning Checklists

Clean and neat are always in style, but cleanliness is imperative when it comes to avoiding germs. Cleaning is necessary before things can be sanitized. Dirt or gross soils will prevent sanitizers and disinfectants from reaching the targeted microbes. Allergens and germs build-up and/or grow in the presence of dirt, dust, and organic materials. Remove shoes at the door to avoid tracking germs and allergens throughout the home. Wipe pets' paws before allowing them to run through the house.

I covered how to apply and how to remove disinfectants in Chapter 2's Defensive Tactics.

Your choice of cleansers and sanitizers or disinfectants is up to you. Always read labels, and choose your weapons based on personal preferences.

Before cleaning sensitive electronics or fabrics, refer to the manufacturers' recommendations for how to clean to avoid fading, bleaching, or otherwise damaging your precious items.

Personal care items such as toothbrushes, orthodontia cases, or contact lens cases should be replaced on a regular basis.

Following this, you will find checklists for various areas of home or workspaces.

Living Room

- o   Disinfect door handles.
- o   Launder removable pillows and covers.
- o   Vacuum and clean upholstered furniture.
- o   Disinfect light switches.
- o   Sanitize remote controls.
- o   Sanitize children's toys.
- o   Wash pet toys.
- o   Clean coasters.
- o   Sanitize cell phones and chargers.
- o   Sanitize computer keyboard, touchscreen, mouse, and mousepad.
- o   Sanitize electronic tablets.
- o   Disinfect landline phones.
- o   Wipe down video games and controllers.
- o   Wipe the covers of DVD's and CD's.
- o   Floors should be vacuumed or swept and mopped.
- o   Consider having carpets cleaned or cleaning carpets yourself.
- o   Dust flat surfaces.
- o   Wash and sanitize trash cans.
- o   Remove cobwebs.
- o   Clean windows, frames, sills, and blinds.

Kitchen

- o   Wipe light switches.
- o   Sanitize door handles.
- o   Disinfect cabinet door handles.
- o   Disinfect drawer pulls.
- o   Wipe down appliance door handles.
- o   Wipe down table and chairs
- o   Sanitize countertops.
- o   Disinfect faucet handles.
- o   Sweep, vacuum, and mop floors where appropriate.
- o   Wash cooking utensils, dishware, and flatware in hot, soapy water.

- o   Sanitize landline phones.
- o   Wash appliance knobs.
- o   Degrease appliance fans and filters.
- o   Wash drip pans.
- o   Dust exhaust fans.
- o   Sanitize cutting boards.
- o   Clean highchairs.
- o   Wash dishcloths and brushes.
- o   Clean the dishwasher inside and out, including the filter or screen.
- o   Sanitize sinks.
- o   Sanitize the sink drain strainer basket and drain plugs.
- o   Wash the processor bowl and blades in hot, soapy water.
- o   Clean out the refrigerator interior, drawers, and racks, and dispose of any questionable foods.
- o   Wash out trash cans and spray with disinfectant spray.
- o   Wash down windows, sills, frames, and blinds.

Bathroom

- o   Disinfect entry door handles.
- o   Sanitize light switches.
- o   Disinfect faucet handles.
- o   Wipe off vanity top.
- o   Sanitize the sink.
- o   Sanitize drawer pulls.
- o   Clean and disinfect the toilet bowl, seat, and rim.
- o   Sanitize the flush handle frequently.
- o   Bidet buttons should be disinfected at least every day.
- o   Towels and wash cloths should be laundered on hottest settings for the fabric.
- o   Towel bars should be dusted.
- o   Toiletry containers, lids, and pump handles should be sanitized like any other contact surface.
- o   The disinfectant spray can needs wiped off, too.
- o   The air freshener can gets handled by every hand in the house at some point.
- o   The candle lighter is another often overlooked contact point.
- o   Tub and shower should be cleaned weekly, or more frequently when someone in the household is ill.
- o   Grab rails should be disinfected regularly.

- o Potty chairs should be sanitized daily; toddlers are not good hand washers.
- o Step stools should be wiped off.
- o Windows, sills, frames, and blinds should be dusted and wiped down.
- o Trash cans should be washed and sanitized.
- o Cobwebs need removed.
- o Floors should be swept, vacuumed, and mopped as needed.

Bedrooms

- o Dust flat surfaces.
- o Sanitize drawer pulls.
- o Wipe down windows, sills, frames, and blinds.
- o Floors should be vacuumed or swept and mopped.
- o Bedding and linens should be laundered once per week, or daily if someone is ill.
- o Clothing should be laundered frequently.
- o Shoes and boots should be wiped outside, removed inside the door, and cleaned before storing.
- o Door handles should be sanitized.
- o Light switches should be disinfected.
- o Remote controls need wiped off.
- o Cell phones and chargers need wiped off because they are one of the most touched items in the home.
- o Tablet or e-reader and charger should be wiped down after use.
- o Trash cans need cleaned and sanitized.
- o Cobwebs must be removed.

Offices

- o Door handles are used by everyone. Disinfect them.
- o Light switches are a high-contact area.
- o Remote controls get frequent use as well.
- o Intercoms see plenty of fingers, also.
- o Phones should be sanitized.
- o Computer, keyboard, mouse, and touchscreen all collect germs from multiple sources.
- o Laser pointers are often shared, and so are the germs that others have left behind.
- o White board markers are a common item and should be sanitized.

- o Desk supplies such as pens, pencils, staplers, calculators, and scissors all need sanitized daily.
- o Copier, printer, or fax keypad and paper drawer pull should be wiped down.
- o Storage and filing cabinet handles must be cleaned.
- o Conference tables and office chairs
- o First-aid cabinet door and latches should be disinfected.
- o Windows, sills, frames, blinds need dusted and wiped.
- o Trash cans should be cleaned and disinfected.

Factory or shop workspaces

- o Wipe down door handles and the frames where they are frequently touched.
- o Time clock keypads and biometric sensors should be disinfected shiftly.
- o Light switches in team rooms or small shops see a lot of hands.
- o Machine touch screens (HMI's) get touched by every operator and break person. Wipe them down with sanitizer.
- o Machine keypads should be wiped off.
- o Tools should be cleaned after use.
- o Toolbox handles and drawer pulls must be cleaned daily.
- o Chairs should be wiped.
- o Desks need dusted.
- o Tables need sanitized.
- o Handrails should be wiped down.
- o Pushbuttons or levers see frequent use and should be disinfected.
- o Pens, pencils, and styluses are touched by a lot of people.
- o Computer, keyboard, mouse, and touchscreen should be cleaned shiftly.
- o Sanitize Lock-out Tag-out boxes and locks, if used.
- o Dry erase markers should be sanitized after use when something is going around.
- o Food contact items should be disinfected per industry standards.
- o Ladders should be cleaned during sanitation.
- o First-aid cabinets' latches should be sanitized like other handles.
- o Broom, squeegee, mop, and dustpan handles get exposed to dirty, contaminated hands and gloves.

- o Phones get hand contact as well as possible saliva while one speaks, then touch one's face. This is extra close contact and should be sanitized frequently.
- o Radios and microphones should be assigned to one person if possible, and they need kept clean.
- o Sanitize intercom buttons.
- o Wipe clipboards.
- o Disinfect the soap dispenser.
- o Do not forget the towel dispenser.
- o Disinfect the bathroom stall doors and latches.
- o Bathroom fixtures, if not cleaned by a service (see bathroom list on previous page), are touched by everyone.
- o The breakroom, if not cleaned by a service, should be cleaned like a kitchen (see list for kitchen on previous page)
- o Locker, latch, and lock should be wiped or sprayed once per week.
- o Floors need scrubbed daily in a high-traffic workspace.

Vehicle

This book is not meant to encompass all there is to clean on a vehicle. I am only concerned with contact surfaces most likely to transfer germs.

- o Door handles should be obvious.
- o Lock or window switches should be wiped weekly on a personal vehicle or daily on a shared vehicle.
- o Push buttons or knobs need cleaned.
- o The signal lever sees a lot of use.
- o The steering wheel is unavoidable as a contact area.
- o Seats are harder to clean, but should be done regularly.
- o Floor mats should be cleaned when you wash the vehicle.
- o Arm rests need cleaned because of sweat and body oils, not just germs.
- o Gear selector/gearshift should be wiped weekly.
- o Wiper controls need cleaned less frequently because of they are not used as often as some other controls.
- o Child safety seats need cleaned regularly. If the child spills drinks or food or otherwise soils the upholstery, clean as soon as possible to avoid growing bacterial and setting permanent stains.
- o Cup holders get grimy in a hurry. Clean spills immediately.
- o Dash and windshield/windows should be dusted and cleaned monthly.

- o The gas door should be wiped whenever the vehicle has been fueled up.
- o The cabin air filter should be changed according to your vehicle's maintenance log or whenever the air smells objectionable.

Public Places

You probably will not be cleaning public places unless that is your job. However, you should keep these contact surfaces in mind to avoid when possible or wash or sanitize hands and personal items as soon as possible after touching. Minimize touching merchandise unless you plan to purchase it. If you choose to wear gloves, disposables are best and should not be reused.

- o Pens
- o Keypads
- o Styluses
- o Checkout belt or counter
- o Service counter or bar
- o Restroom doors, dispensers, and dryers
- o Manual doors
- o Cooler or freezer handles
- o Restaurant counters, tables, chairs, dispensers
- o Money
- o Carts
- o Handshakes
- o Mobility aids (rails, scooters)
- o Handrails
- o Elevator buttons
- o Clipboards
- o Waiting room furniture and magazines
- o Playground or sports equipment
- o Picnic tables, grills
- o Water fountains
- o Fuel pumps
- o ATM's

Appendix D

Preparedness Supplies

Preparedness is a topic that can take up multiple volumes by itself. For the purposes of this book, I will concentrate on supplies that will come in handy when illness, parasites, and injury are your primary concerns. No matter what the disaster, some things are important to have on hand. A month of supplies should be the minimum if you have space to store them and can afford to acquire said supplies. I realize not everyone can afford the basics, let alone stockpiling them. Prioritize by deciding what is most necessary in an anticipated situation.

Home

If you are sheltering in place during an epidemic, or if a storm has temporarily left you without power, some basic tips and techniques will avoid a minor inconvenience from becoming a life-threatening health emergency.

- o N-95 masks are useful if someone is sick. The sick person should wear one to avoid spreading germs unless wearing a mask hinders breathing. Regular dust masks or cloth masks may be better than nothing for particulates or allergens, but they probably will not be able to filter out microbes. Still, any mask can reduce the number of germs sneezed or coughed out by a sick individual.
- o Cleaning supplies, whatever ones you prefer to use, are extremely important. At the bare minimum, keep two extra cans or bottles of each cleaner (or the ingredients for your home-made cleaners), on hand. Try to stick with ready-to-use cleaners rather than ones that must be diluted in case water supply is an issue.
- o Rotate stock using FIFO, or First In, First Out. Whether you are referring to food supplies, cleaning supplies, or personal hygiene supplies, rotate the items so that the oldest one is in front and gets used first.
- o Non-perishable foods are the best to keep around in case you cannot get to the store or the store shelves are empty. Stock up

on what you eat most often. 20 cans of spinach will not keep anyone from starving if they gag when they try to eat it. Canned foods also contain some water, which can be a life saver if the water supply is uncertain.

- Stock up on ready-to-eat soups rather than condensed in case water supply is a problem.
- Personal hygiene products should be stocked so that there is at least one extra in the cabinet, if possible. Do not worry about cosmetics; concern yourself with toothpaste, shampoo, soaps, contact lens solution, deodorant. Keeping a pair of prescription glasses around can reduce or eliminate the need for contact solution. Makeup is not essential, so do not waste precious funds on it.
- Keep a pair of prescription glasses in each vehicle in case you lose a contact or break your regular glasses. Even an old prescription may keep you navigating safely.
- A first aid kit is essential, but most kits sold to the general public are only equipped for a minor scrape or headache. Gradually put together a kit that fits your lifestyle and the injuries you are likely to encounter during your activities. For example, if you are a mountain biker, ace bandages, triple-antibiotic ointment, gauze, first-aid tape, and cold packs would be good for you to keep on hand at home or in a backpack.
- Water filters, such as those marketed to hikers, could be important if the water supply is compromised.
- If water safety is questionable and filters are unavailable, boil water for a minimum of five minutes. If you spend a lot of time in the outdoors, learning ways of finding safe water could be the difference between life and death.
- Fresh water is imperative. If you can buy drinking water, then stockpile as much as you can. Plan on a gallon of water per person per day. Rotate the stock by FIFO.
- Stock up on infant formula, if used.
- If you have lost power, avoid opening the refrigerator or freezer unless absolutely necessary. If the outside temperature is below 40° F. consider putting perishables outside if this can be done without fear of tampering or theft. An enclosed porch, shed, or garage will be safer than just setting it outside. Alternatively,

you can use snow or icicles in coolers or containers frozen outside to cool the items in your refrigerator or freezer.

o In case of a power outage, use up perishables first.

o Prescription medications are the hardest thing to stockpile; there are strict laws on how much can be dispensed. The best one can do is try to avoid running out of them. During the COVID-19 pandemic of 2020, which is happening as I write this, pharmacies and pharmaceutical manufacturers are among the businesses considered essential, so they have been permitted to continue operations.

o Consumable household supplies such as toilet paper, facial tissues, and paper towels are hard to come by when panicky shoppers wipe out store inventories. Figure out how much of these your family go through in a month so you can keep ample supplies on hand. Do not forget to include tampons, pads, bladder control products, diapers, and baby wipes in these supplies. Washable handkerchiefs, towels, and diapers are a lot eco-friendlier than disposables, but washing them may not be practical, depending on the health of the members of the household or water quality issues. Also, disposable items may be safer for the caregivers of sick persons.

o Paper plates, paper cups and disposable eating utensils may be best when feeding contagious patients. Keeping some on hand can also be helpful if potable water is in short supply.

o Laundry detergent and liquid fabric softener are nice to stock up on, but they are not true necessities. Obviously, detergent can be used to clean clothes, dishcloths, bath towels, bedding, handkerchiefs, cloth diapers, and so on, but the biggest germ-killing effect of doing laundry is the temperature. Use the hottest temperature the fabrics can endure in both the washer and dryer, if used. I specified liquid fabric softener for two reasons: 1. Weather permitting, hanging laundry outside where possible allows the sun's UV rays to do the disinfecting effectively for free. 2. If there is a power outage that precludes use of the dryer, you still get better-smelling laundry than you would without softener. Hanging laundry outside is not a good idea for someone with severe allergies to pollen or other outdoor triggers.

o   Grow your own food as much as you can. This alone will help prevent the transmission of contagious diseases by eliminating the need to go to the store as often. If you have a window and room for a flowerpot, you have room to grow something edible. A window planter full of leaf lettuce, a bucket with a tomato plant in it, a flower bed with radishes and nasturtiums, a patio with pots containing carrots or strawberries, or a full-sized garden and orchard. Grow whatever you can where you can. Eat it fresh, freeze the harvest, or home-can the bounty; every little bit helps reduce your reliance on outside sources. Gardening itself has mental and physical health benefits, the extra food inventory will supplement or replace store-bought groceries, the nutritional quality of the food will likely surpass that from commercial growers, and the taste is almost always superior to anything you can buy from commercial suppliers. Growing your own food is also environmentally friendly because you reduce your carbon footprint by lessening the demand for food to be transported.

o   Remember to stock up for your pets as well. Pine shavings, feed, water, hay, straw, and all of your usual supplies will still be needed. Always keep extra in stock for your animals the same as you would for your family.

o   Firearms and ammunition are valid ways of protecting your family from looters, for protecting your livestock or family from predators or diseased animals, and for hunting or slaughtering animals if an extended food shortage should develop. Regardless of your feelings about firearms, learning to handle them safely can provide peace of mind and make you better able to adapt to any situation.

Vehicle

Many of us spend a good portion of our days commuting. A backpack with some basics in it can travel with you, even on public transportation. "Bug-out-bags" can be purchased as a kit or put together on your own for a custom stash of things you may need. They are geared more to survival situations, so I will leave the bug-out-bag discussion for another day. Keep in mind, a bug-out-bag may also contain items that would be illegal to carry everywhere with you. Here, I will concentrate on our prevailing topic of avoiding infectious diseases.

- Travel-sized packs of baby wipes are good for your backpack because you will often be out-and-about with nowhere to wash your hands.
- Hand sanitizer in a travel size can fit into your backpack or be clipped on. A larger sized bottle of the germ killer is nice to have on hand in the car for after you have pumped fuel or touched shopping carts. I recommend alcohol-based sanitizers because those containing triclosan carry some potential for adverse health effects. Side-note: triclosan is in a lot more products than just hand sanitizer. Studies are ongoing.
- A full water bottle, reusable or disposable, is good to carry regardless of where you are going. Whether you need to drink it or wash with it, it should be considered indispensable.
- A vehicle first-aid kit with at least two pairs of exam gloves and some cut-resistant gloves, antiseptic, and bandages is a good start. For your backpack, I would at least include the exam and cut resistant kinds of gloves.
- A container of disinfecting wipes can be used to quickly sanitize your door handles, steering wheel, gear shift, and controls on the go. Be careful about getting them on upholstery or carpet; some of them will bleach porous materials.
- Carry your own ink pen so you will not need to use the pens at the doctor's office or bank.

Appendix E

Personal Hygiene

In terms of avoiding contagious diseases, few practices can be more effective than good personal hygiene.

- o Shower or bathe daily. Showering is preferable because one does not sit in his own filth.
- o Showering before bed is beneficial for removing any hitchhiking germs or allergens that would otherwise be carried to bed with you.
- o Wash least dirty areas first and progress to dirtier areas. Wash and rinse hair with shampoo. Then wash the face and hands. Next wash the torso, arms, and legs. Armpits and genitals are next. Feet get washed last. Rinse thoroughly before toweling dry.
- o Any bar soap will do for washing the body. If you prefer body wash, replace the pouf regularly.
- o Anti-perspirants and deodorants for underarms can be chosen by personal preference. Deodorants will need to be reapplied more often to prevent the growth of bacteria, which is what causes body odor.
- o Floss at least once per day, preferably before bedtime. Flossing is the best way to remove food particles and plaque from tooth surfaces between teeth and below the gum line. Neglecting these areas allows bacteria to form colonies, which reach harmful levels in about three months. Such an infection can lead to dental caries (cavities), gum disease (gingivitis), or bone deterioration (periodontal disease.)
- o Brush teeth after each meal according to the directions on your chosen toothpaste. Do not swallow toothpaste.
- o Rinse with water or an antiseptic mouthwash, swishing between teeth to flush the loosened debris away and kill germs that cause bad breath and infection. Spit all of it out.

Appendix F

Proper Use of Gloves

It is common knowledge that gloves are ubiquitous PPE (personal protective equipment) when it comes to avoiding contagions.

Choose the right gloves for the job. There is a glove for just about any task. Here, I will stick to avoiding pathogens.

Cut-resistant gloves can prevent scrapes or cuts from damaging the skin and opening a pathway for infectious agents to enter the body.

Exam gloves are higher density materials than disposable cleaning gloves. The cheap ones will tear too easily to be relied on for PPE from infection. Exam gloves are usually offered in latex or nitrile materials, the latter being for those who may be allergic to latex.

Latex or rubber gloves are usually used for cleaning. Cleaning gloves, or rubber gloves, are a heavier barrier for use with chemicals and soaps to avoid damage to the skin or absorption of the chemicals through the skin.

To minimize the chances of carrying germs from one area to another, clean the less contaminated areas first. The mirror is less germy than the vanity, which is less germ-ridden than the sink, which is less germ-loaded than the toilet. It is best to dispose of rubber gloves after use, but if you must reuse them, wash your hands with the gloves still on. Rinse them off, then hang them somewhere to air dry. Then wash your hands again.

Never use the bathroom gloves in any other area.

All of your precautions will be for naught if you touch the outside of the gloves when removing them and get the microbes on your hands. Keep reading for the proper way to remove gloves.

- o Pinch the cuff of one glove with the index finger and thumb of the other gloved hand. Peel the glove off, inside-out, keeping hold of the removed glove with the still-gloved hand. Slip the fingers of the bare hand inside the cuff of the other glove so it can be peeled off, inside-out, and disposed of. This method will avoid contact with the outside, contaminated surface of the gloves. Discard disposable gloves in the garbage or in a biohazard bag.
- o Wash your hands thoroughly.

Acknowledgements

Thank you, Traci Butler, for never saying never and supporting my ideas, no matter how crazy they sound.

Thanks to my kids, Kevin Dillon and Ashley Dillon, for never saying what you really think about my next project idea.

I would like to thank Rick Schumaker for being my "farmhand" and freeing up my time to write as well as sending me to my office to work.

About the Author

Goldie Kirkbride is an Ohio native who would not have it any other way. She spent three years living in Florida but decided Ohio would always be home.

Growing up poor, she learned the difference between necessities and luxuries, which translates into common sense and practicality that have enabled her to conquer every challenge that has come her way.

School was a window to the world for Goldie, and she has never lost her desire to learn. Since graduating high school, she has completed several courses of study:

ICS School of Automotive Mechanics

WCSCC Adult Educational Classes in Pneumatics and in Basic Electricity

Stratford Institute Creative Writing School

International Institute of Nutrition Certified Health Coach

Goldie has also worked in production in various manufacturing facilities including two food processing plants.

For over two decades, Goldie has volunteered for first-aid responder roles, which require continual recertification in First Aid, AED, and CPR. She was also a leading proponent for fire-extinguisher training for key plant technicians at the world's largest jam and jelly factory, where she still works as a Level 10 Technician, which is a leadership role with equipment maintenance and personnel training responsibilities.

Currently, Goldie lives on seven acres in northeast Ohio with a menagerie of animals including chickens, dogs, cats, a guinea, and a horse. In her spare time, she writes, spends time with her animals, gardens, preserves the extra food, and coaches friends and family on health goals, pro bono. She has two children, two grandchildren, and another on the way.

Miss Kirkbride has never lost her thirst for knowledge. She is passionate about helping others find natural ways to reach their health goals and encourages gardening as a means of feeding people the most nutritious way possible.

Look for the next book in the Practical Living Series: Practical Adulting: Tips for Life After High School.

www.ingramcontent.com/pod-product-compliance
Lightning Source LLC
Chambersburg PA
CBHW051422250726
48655CB00003B/1188